Nutrition for Expectant Mothers

Optimizing nutrition during pregnancy for a healthy baby

BY LORENA SMITH

TABLE OF CONTENTS

Introduction

Congratulations, you're pregnant! As an expectant mother, you likely have a lot on your mind, from preparing for your baby's arrival to ensuring a healthy pregnancy. One of the most important things you can do for your growing baby is to provide them with the nutrients they need to thrive.

Pregnancy is a time of incredible change, both for your body and your baby's. From the moment of conception, your body is working hard to create a safe and nourishing environment for your little one to grow and develop. Proper nutrition during pregnancy is essential for supporting fetal growth and development, reducing the risk of pregnancy complications, and ensuring your own health and well-being.

As you embark on this exciting journey, you may have questions about what to eat, how much to eat, and which nutrients are essential for a healthy pregnancy. You may also be wondering how to manage common pregnancy-related symptoms such as morning sickness, fatigue, and heartburn.

In this book, we'll explore the fundamentals of pregnancy nutrition, from the key nutrients needed for fetal development to the foods to eat and avoid during pregnancy. We'll cover the basics of building a healthy plate and optimizing portion sizes, as well as providing sample meals and snacks for pregnant women. We'll also delve into the vitamins and minerals that are essential for a healthy pregnancy, including their recommended daily intake and food sources.

But we won't stop there. Pregnancy is a time of many changes, both physical and emotional, and we'll be with you every step of the way. We'll share practical strategies for managing common pregnancy-related symptoms with nutrition, including dealing with food aversions and cravings. We'll also address special considerations for women with high-risk pregnancies, including gestational diabetes, hypertension, and other conditions.

And, once your baby arrives, we'll provide guidance on postpartum nutrition for a healthy recovery and successful breastfeeding. We'll discuss strategies for maintaining a healthy weight and balanced diet post-pregnancy, as well as the importance of continuing to prioritize your own health and well-being as a new mother.

Whether you're a first-time mom or a seasoned pro, this book is designed to be your go-to guide for navigating the often-confusing world of pregnancy nutrition. We'll break down the science behind optimal nutrition during pregnancy and translate it into practical tips and advice that you can apply to your daily life. So sit back, relax, and let's dive into the world of pregnancy nutrition together!

CHAPTER 1

Introduction to Pregnancy Nutrition

Congratulations on your pregnancy! This is a very exciting time in your life, and as an expectant mother, you are likely concerned about the health and well-being of both you and your growing baby. One of the most important things you can do to ensure a healthy pregnancy is to pay close attention to your nutrition.

Nutrition plays a crucial role in the development of your baby, and it can also have a significant impact on your own health during pregnancy. Eating a well-balanced diet with a variety of nutrients can help to prevent complications such as gestational diabetes, pre-eclampsia, and premature birth.

In this chapter, we will discuss the basics of pregnancy nutrition, including the nutrients you need, the foods you should eat, and the ones you should avoid. We will also touch on the importance of maintaining a healthy weight during pregnancy and the potential consequences of gaining too much or too little weight.

Throughout your pregnancy, it is important to remember that every woman and every pregnancy is unique. Your specific nutritional needs may differ from someone else's based on factors such as your age, weight, and medical history. Therefore, it is always a good idea to consult with your healthcare provider before making any significant changes to your diet.

With that said, let's dive into the basics of pregnancy nutrition and start preparing your body for a healthy pregnancy and a healthy baby.

Importance of proper nutrition during pregnancy

Proper nutrition during pregnancy is critical for both the mother and the developing fetus. The fetus depends entirely on the mother for nutrients, and inadequate or imbalanced nutrition can result in significant health problems for both the mother and the baby.

One of the most important reasons for proper nutrition during pregnancy is to support the growth and development of the fetus. The nutrients provided by the mother are essential for the formation of the fetal brain, organs, bones, and other tissues. Inadequate nutrition during this critical period can result in low birth weight, which is associated with increased risk of infant mortality, developmental delays, and chronic diseases later in life.

Proper nutrition during pregnancy can also help to reduce the risk of complications such as gestational diabetes and pre-eclampsia. Gestational diabetes occurs when the mother's blood sugar levels become too high during pregnancy, and it can lead to complications such as high birth weight, respiratory distress, and low blood sugar in the baby. Pre-eclampsia is a serious condition that can cause high blood pressure, protein in the urine, and damage to the mother's organs. It can also increase the risk of premature birth and other complications.

In addition to supporting fetal growth and development and reducing the risk of complications, proper nutrition during pregnancy can also help the mother maintain her own health. Adequate intake of nutrients such as iron, folic acid, and calcium can help prevent anemia, neural tube defects, and bone loss, respectively. Eating a healthy diet during pregnancy can also help to maintain a healthy weight and reduce the risk of excess weight gain, which can lead to complications such as gestational diabetes, pre-eclampsia, and cesarean delivery.

Overall, proper nutrition during pregnancy is essential for the health and well-being of both the mother and the developing fetus.

Key nutrients needed for fetal development

There are several key nutrients that are essential for fetal development and that should be included in a healthy pregnancy diet. These include:

- Folic acid: Folic acid is important for the development of the neural tube, which forms the baby's brain and spinal cord. Adequate intake of folic acid can help prevent neural tube defects such as spina bifida. Good sources of folic acid include leafy green vegetables, beans, fortified cereals, and citrus fruits.

- Iron: Iron is necessary for the production of hemoglobin, which carries oxygen to the baby's cells. Iron deficiency during pregnancy can lead to anemia, which can cause fatigue, weakness, and other complications. Good sources of iron include lean meats, beans, fortified cereals, and dark leafy green vegetables.

- Calcium: Calcium is essential for the development of the baby's bones and teeth. Adequate intake of calcium during pregnancy can also help prevent bone loss in the mother. Good sources of calcium include dairy products, fortified juices and cereals, and leafy green vegetables.

- Vitamin D: Vitamin D is important for the absorption of calcium and for the development of the baby's bones and teeth. Good sources of vitamin D include fortified milk and cereals, fatty fish, and exposure to sunlight.

- Omega-3 fatty acids: Omega-3 fatty acids are important for the development of the baby's brain and eyes. Good sources of omega-3 fatty acids include fatty fish, such as salmon and sardines, and walnuts.

In addition to these key nutrients, it is important to eat a variety of fruits, vegetables, whole grains, and lean proteins to ensure adequate intake of all necessary nutrients.

Risks associated with poor nutrition during pregnancy

Poor nutrition during pregnancy can have serious consequences for both the mother and the developing fetus. Some of the potential risks associated with poor nutrition during pregnancy include:

- Low birth weight: Inadequate intake of nutrients during pregnancy can result in low birth weight, which is associated with increased risk of infant mortality, developmental delays, and chronic diseases later in life.

- Neural tube defects: Inadequate intake of folic acid during pregnancy can increase the risk of neural tube defects such as spina bifida.

- Anemia: Iron deficiency during pregnancy can lead to anemia, which can cause fatigue, weakness, and other complications.

- Pre-eclampsia: Poor nutrition during pregnancy can increase the risk of pre-eclampsia, a serious condition that can cause high blood pressure, protein in the urine, and damage to the mother's organs.

- Gestational diabetes: Inadequate intake of nutrients during pregnancy can increase the risk of gestational diabetes, which can lead to complications such as high birth weight, respiratory distress, and low blood sugar in the baby.

- Premature birth: Poor nutrition during pregnancy can increase the risk of premature birth, which can lead to a range of complications for the baby including respiratory distress, developmental delays, and long-term disabilities.

- Behavioral problems: Poor nutrition during pregnancy has been linked to an increased risk of behavioral problems in children, including attention deficit hyperactivity disorder (ADHD).

It is important to note that the risks associated with poor nutrition during pregnancy can be mitigated by making changes to the diet and/or taking supplements to ensure adequate intake of all necessary nutrients. Pregnant women should aim to eat a balanced diet that includes a variety of fruits, vegetables, whole grains, and lean proteins, and should work with their healthcare provider to ensure that they are meeting their nutritional needs.

Conclusion:

Proper nutrition during pregnancy is essential for the health and well-being of both the mother and the developing fetus. Adequate intake of key nutrients such as folic acid, iron, calcium, and protein is crucial for fetal growth and development, and can help prevent a range of complications including low birth weight, neural tube defects, anemia, pre-eclampsia, gestational diabetes, premature birth, and behavioral problems in children.

On the other hand, poor nutrition during pregnancy can have serious consequences for both the mother and the baby, increasing the risk of a range of complications and long-term health issues. It is important for expectant mothers to understand the importance of proper nutrition during pregnancy and to work with their healthcare provider to ensure that they are meeting their nutritional needs.

In the following chapters, we will explore in detail the key nutrients needed for fetal development, the foods that are rich in these nutrients, and practical tips for maintaining a healthy diet during pregnancy. By following these guidelines, expectant mothers can help ensure a healthy pregnancy and give their babies the best possible start in life.

CHAPTER 2

Buulding a Healthy Plate

Pregnancy is a time when a woman's body requires additional nutrients to support the growth and development of the fetus. A balanced and healthy diet is essential to ensure that both the mother and the baby receive the necessary nutrients. Building a healthy plate involves selecting foods from different food groups in appropriate portion sizes. In this chapter, we will discuss the food groups and their importance during pregnancy, optimal portion sizes, and sample meals and snacks for pregnant women.

Food Groups and Their Importance During Pregnancy

During pregnancy, it is important for women to consume a well-balanced diet that provides all the necessary nutrients for both themselves and their developing baby. This can be achieved by eating a variety of foods from different food groups, including fruits and vegetables, whole grains, protein, dairy, and healthy fats. Each of these food groups plays a unique and important role in supporting the growth and development of the fetus.

•Fruits and Vegetables

Fruits and vegetables are a rich source of vitamins, minerals, fiber, and antioxidants, which are important for the health of the mother and the baby. These nutrients help to reduce the risk of pregnancy complications, such as pre-eclampsia and gestational diabetes, and promote healthy fetal development. Fruits and vegetables are also low in calories and high in water content, which can help to prevent excessive weight gain during pregnancy. Examples of fruits that are particularly beneficial during pregnancy include oranges, strawberries, kiwis, and grapefruits, which are high in vitamin C. Dark leafy greens, such as spinach, kale, and broccoli, are also good sources of folate, iron, and calcium, which are important for fetal development.

•Whole Grains

Whole grains are a good source of complex carbohydrates, fiber, and B vitamins, which are essential for the health of the mother and the baby. Complex carbohydrates provide a steady supply of energy, while fiber helps to prevent constipation and promote healthy digestion. B vitamins, such as thiamine, riboflavin, and niacin, are important for fetal brain and nervous system development. Examples of whole grains that are particularly beneficial during pregnancy include oatmeal, brown rice, and whole wheat bread.

•Protein

Protein is essential for the growth and development of the baby, as it helps to build and repair tissues, produce enzymes and hormones, and transport nutrients throughout the body. Pregnant women should aim to consume at least 2-3 servings of protein daily, including lean meats, poultry, fish, beans, lentils, and tofu. It is important to choose lean sources of protein, as high-fat meats can increase the risk of excessive weight gain and other pregnancy complications.

•Dairy

Dairy products are a rich source of calcium, which is important for the development of the baby's bones and teeth. Calcium also plays a role in blood clotting, muscle function, and nerve function. Examples include milk, yogurt, and cheese. Low-fat or non-fat dairy products are preferred, as they are lower in saturated fat.

•Healthy Fats

Healthy fats, such as those found in nuts, seeds, avocado, and fatty fish, are important for the development of the baby's brain and nervous system. Omega-3 fatty acids, in particular, are essential for fetal brain development and may help to reduce the risk of preterm labor and postpartum depression.
Examples of healthy fats that are particularly beneficial during pregnancy include salmon, tuna, walnuts, flaxseed, chia seeds, and avocado. It is important to limit the consumption of high-fat foods that are low in

nutrients, such as fried foods, processed snacks, and sweets.

In conclusion, consuming a well-balanced diet that includes a variety of foods from different food groups is essential for the health of both the mother and the baby during pregnancy.

Optimal portion sizes

When it comes to healthy eating during pregnancy, it's important to not only choose nutrient-rich foods but also pay attention to portion sizes. Eating the appropriate portion sizes can help pregnant women avoid excessive weight gain, which can increase the risk of complications during pregnancy and delivery.

The American College of Obstetricians and Gynecologists (ACOG) recommends that pregnant women consume an additional 340 calories per day during the second trimester and an additional 450 calories per day during the third trimester. However, calorie requirements can vary depending on a woman's pre-pregnancy weight, height, age, and activity level. Therefore, it's important for pregnant women to work with their healthcare provider or a registered dietitian to determine their individual calorie needs.

In addition to calorie needs, pregnant women should aim to consume a balanced diet that includes foods from different food groups in appropriate portion sizes. The following are some guidelines for optimal portion sizes during pregnancy:

- Fruits and Vegetables: Pregnant women should aim to consume at least 2-3 servings of fruits and 3-4 servings of vegetables daily. A serving of fruits or vegetables is typically 1 cup of raw leafy greens or 1/2 cup of cooked or raw vegetables or fruits. To ensure variety, pregnant women should try to consume different colors and types of fruits and vegetables.

- Whole Grains: Whole grains are a good source of complex carbohydrates, fiber, and B vitamins. Pregnant women should aim to consume at least 6-8 servings of whole grains daily, including bread, cereal, rice, pasta, and quinoa. A serving of whole grains is typically 1 slice of bread, 1/2 cup of cooked rice or pasta, or 1 ounce of dry cereal.

- Protein: Protein is essential for the growth and development of the baby. Pregnant women should aim to consume at least 2-3 servings of protein daily, including lean meats, poultry, fish, beans, lentils, and tofu. A serving of protein is typically 3-4 ounces of meat, fish, or poultry, 1/2 cup of cooked beans or lentils, or 2 tablespoons of nut butter.

- Dairy: Dairy products are rich in calcium, which is important for the development of the baby's bones and teeth. Pregnant women should aim to consume at least 3-4 servings of dairy daily, including milk, yogurt, and cheese. A serving of dairy is typically 1 cup of milk or yogurt or 1.5 ounces of cheese.

- Fats: Healthy fats such as those found in nuts, seeds, avocado, and fatty fish are important for the development of the baby's brain and nervous system. Pregnant women should aim to consume 2-3 servings of healthy fats daily. A serving of healthy fats is typically 1/4 cup of nuts or seeds, 1/2 avocado, or 3-4 ounces of fatty fish.

It's important for pregnant women to avoid overeating, especially high-calorie, low-nutrient foods such as sweets, fast food, and processed snacks. Instead, they should aim for a balanced plate with 50% fruits and vegetables, 25% whole grains, and 25% protein. Pregnant women should also listen to their hunger and fullness cues and eat when hungry and stop when satisfied.

Pregnant women should also pay attention to their fluid intake. The recommended daily fluid intake during pregnancy is 10 cups (80 ounces) of water, which includes fluids from foods and beverages. Pregnant women should aim to drink water throughout the day and avoid sugary or caffeinated beverages.

In summary, optimal portion sizes during pregnancy involve consuming a balanced diet that includes foods from different food groups in appropriate amounts. Pregnant women should aim to consume enough calories to support the growth and development of their baby but avoid excessive weight gain by paying attention to their portion sizes. A balanced plate should consist of 50% fruits and vegetables, 25% whole grains, and 25% protein, along with healthy fats in appropriate amounts. Pregnant women should also listen to their hunger and fullness cues and drink enough water throughout the day.

In addition to following these general guidelines, pregnant women should work with their healthcare provider or a registered dietitian to determine their individual nutrition needs and create a personalized meal plan. A registered dietitian can also provide education on appropriate portion sizes and help pregnant women make healthy food choices that meet their individual needs.

It's also important to note that pregnant women may experience food aversions or cravings, which can make it challenging to follow a balanced diet. In such cases, it's important to be flexible and find healthy alternatives that still meet their nutritional needs.

<u>Conclusion:</u>

In conclusion, building a healthy plate during pregnancy is crucial for the proper growth and development of the fetus. A healthy pregnancy diet should include a variety of nutrient-dense foods from each food group, such as whole grains, fruits and vegetables, lean proteins, and healthy fats. It is also important to consume adequate amounts of key nutrients, such as folic acid, iron, and calcium, to support the growth and development of the fetus. By incorporating a variety of healthy foods into their meals and snacks, pregnant women can help ensure that they are providing their growing baby with the essential nutrients they need to thrive.

CHAPTER 3

Foods to Eat and Avoid

Pregnancy is a critical time when expectant mothers need to pay close attention to their diet to ensure optimal nutrition for themselves and their developing babies. In this chapter, we will discuss the foods to eat and avoid during pregnancy, as well as important food safety considerations.

Foods to Focus on During Pregnancy for Optimal Nutrition

During pregnancy, the body undergoes a range of changes to support fetal growth and development, and it is important to consume a balanced and nutrient-dense diet to meet the increased demands of the body. Consuming a variety of foods from all food groups can help ensure a range of vitamins, minerals, and other nutrients that are essential for fetal development and maternal health.

1. Fruits and Vegetables

Fruits and vegetables are an important source of vitamins, minerals, and fiber that are essential for fetal growth and development. These foods are also low in calories and high in water content, which can help prevent constipation and promote healthy digestion during pregnancy. Eating a variety of fruits and vegetables of different colors can help ensure a range of nutrients, such as:

•Vitamin C: This vitamin is important for fetal growth and development, and can help support a healthy immune system. Foods rich in vitamin C include citrus fruits, kiwi, strawberries, tomatoes, and bell peppers.

•Folate: This B vitamin is important for fetal neural tube development, and can help prevent birth defects. Foods rich in folate include leafy green vegetables, citrus fruits, legumes, and fortified cereals.

•Vitamin A: This vitamin is important for fetal development, particularly for the eyes, skin, and immune system. Foods rich in vitamin A include carrots, sweet potatoes, spinach, and cantaloupe.

•Potassium: This mineral is important for maintaining healthy blood pressure and can help prevent pre-eclampsia during pregnancy. Foods rich in potassium include bananas, avocados, tomatoes, and spinach.

2. Lean Proteins

Protein is an essential nutrient that is important for fetal growth and development, as well as for maternal health. During pregnancy, the body needs more protein to support the growth of the placenta and the developing fetus. Good sources of lean protein include:

•Poultry: Chicken and turkey are good sources of lean protein, and are also rich in iron and zinc that are essential for fetal growth and development.

•Fish: Fish is an important source of omega-3 fatty acids, which are important for fetal brain development. Choose low-mercury fish such as salmon, sardines, and trout.

•Eggs: Eggs are a good source of protein and also contain choline, which is important for fetal brain development.

•Beans and Legumes: Beans and legumes are a good source of plant-based protein, and also contain fiber, iron, and folate that are important for fetal growth and development.

3. Whole Grains

Whole grains such as brown rice, quinoa, and whole wheat bread are an important source of fiber, vitamins, and minerals that are essential for fetal growth and development. These foods can also help regulate blood sugar levels and prevent constipation during pregnancy. Good sources of whole grains include:

•Brown Rice: Brown rice is a good source of fiber, magnesium, and selenium, and can also help regulate blood sugar levels.

•Quinoa: Quinoa is a good source of protein, fiber, and iron, and can be used as a substitute for rice or pasta.

•Whole Wheat Bread: Whole wheat bread is a good source of fiber and B vitamins, and can be used as a healthy alternative to white bread.

4. Dairy Products

Dairy products such as milk, cheese, and yogurt are important sources of calcium and other nutrients that are essential for fetal bone development. Calcium is also important for maintaining healthy blood pressure during pregnancy. Good sources of dairy products include:

•Milk: Milk is a good source of calcium and vitamin D, and can also be fortified with other nutrients such as iron.

•Cheese: Cheese is a good source of calcium and protein, but should be consumed in moderation due to its high calorie content. Hard cheese, such as cheddar or parmesan, is a better choice than soft cheese, such as brie or feta, as it is less likely to contain harmful bacteria.

•Yogurt: Yogurt is a good source of calcium and protein, and also contains probiotics that can help support a healthy gut.

Foods and drinks to avoid or limit during pregnancy

While it is important to focus on consuming a nutrient-dense diet during pregnancy, there are also foods and drinks that should be avoided or limited to reduce the risk of harm to the developing fetus.

- Fish with high levels of mercury: Some types of fish contain high levels of mercury, which can harm the developing nervous system of the fetus. Pregnant women should avoid fish with high levels of mercury, such as shark, swordfish, king mackerel, and tilefish. Instead, they can opt for fish with low levels of mercury, such as salmon, canned light tuna, and shrimp.

- Processed foods: Processed foods are often high in salt, sugar, and unhealthy fats, and are generally low in nutrients. Pregnant women should limit their consumption of processed foods and instead opt for fresh, whole foods that are high in nutrients.

- Artificial sweeteners: Some artificial sweeteners, such as saccharin, should be avoided during pregnancy. Other sweeteners, such as aspartame, are generally considered safe in moderation, but pregnant women should consult with their healthcare provider before consuming them.

- Unwashed produce: Unwashed fruits and vegetables can be contaminated with harmful bacteria and parasites, which can cause foodborne illness. Pregnant women should always wash their produce thoroughly before eating.

- Deli meats: Deli meats can be contaminated with harmful bacteria and should be avoided during pregnancy, or at least heated to a safe internal temperature before consuming.

- Raw sprouts: Raw sprouts, such as alfalfa and clover, can be contaminated with harmful bacteria and should be avoided during pregnancy.

Food Safety Considerations

In addition to avoiding certain foods and drinks during pregnancy, it is important to take other food safety precautions to reduce the risk of foodborne illness. These precautions include:

- Avoiding unpasteurized juice and cider: Unpasteurized juice and cider can contain harmful bacteria and should be avoided during pregnancy.

- Choosing pasteurized dairy products: Unpasteurized dairy products, such as raw milk and certain cheeses, can contain harmful bacteria that can cause foodborne illness. It is recommended to choose pasteurized dairy products during pregnancy.

- Washing hands and surfaces: Hands and surfaces should be washed thoroughly before and after preparing food, particularly raw meat, poultry, and fish.

- Storing food properly: Food should be stored at the correct temperature to prevent the growth of harmful bacteria. Raw meat, poultry, and fish should be stored separately from ready-to-eat foods to reduce the risk of cross-contamination.

- Using safe cooking methods: Meat, poultry, and fish should be cooked to a safe internal temperature to reduce the risk of foodborne illness.

- Avoiding food that has been left out at room temperature: Food that has been left out at room temperature for more than two hours can become contaminated with harmful bacteria and should be avoided during pregnancy.

Conclusion:

Pregnancy is a critical time to focus on a nutrient-dense diet and to avoid certain foods and drinks that can be harmful to the developing fetus. Foods and drinks to avoid or limit during pregnancy include fish with high levels of mercury, processed foods, artificial sweeteners, unwashed produce, deli meats, and raw sprouts. Additionally, taking food safety precautions is essential to reduce the risk of foodborne illness. These precautions include avoiding unpasteurized juice and cider, choosing pasteurized dairy products, washing hands and surfaces, storing food properly, using safe cooking methods, and avoiding food that has been left out at room temperature. By following these guidelines, expectant mothers can help support a healthy pregnancy and give their babies the best possible start in life.

CHAPTER 4

Vitamins and Minerals for Pregnancy

As an expectant mother, it is essential to ensure that your body is getting all the necessary vitamins and minerals for a healthy pregnancy. During pregnancy, your body's requirements for certain nutrients increase significantly, and a deficiency in any of these nutrients can have serious consequences for both you and your baby.

In this chapter, we will discuss the essential vitamins and minerals for a healthy pregnancy, their recommended daily intake, and food sources. We will also touch on the role of prenatal supplements and how they can help to meet your body's nutritional needs during pregnancy.

Essential Vitamins for a Healthy Pregnancy

Vitamins are organic compounds that are essential for the normal growth and development of the body. They are required in small amounts, but their deficiency can cause severe health problems. During pregnancy, the body's requirements for certain vitamins increase significantly, and it is essential to ensure that you are getting enough of these vitamins to support a healthy pregnancy.

1.   Folic Acid (Vitamin B9)

Folic acid is a B vitamin that is crucial for the development of the neural tube, which forms the baby's brain and spinal cord. The neural tube develops during the first month of pregnancy, so it is recommended that women take 400-800 micrograms (mcg) of folic acid daily, ideally starting before pregnancy and continuing through the first trimester.

A deficiency in folic acid during pregnancy can lead to neural tube defects such as spina bifida or anencephaly. Neural tube defects are serious birth defects that can affect the baby's brain and spinal cord. Therefore, it is essential to ensure that you are getting enough folic acid in your diet or through supplements.

Food sources of folic acid include leafy greens, citrus fruits, beans, and fortified cereals. However, it can be challenging to get enough folic acid from food alone, so supplements are often recommended. Many prenatal vitamins contain the recommended amount of folic acid, so it is essential to choose a supplement specifically designed for pregnancy and to consult with your healthcare provider before starting any new supplement regimen.

2.   Vitamin D

Vitamin D is a fat-soluble vitamin that helps the body absorb calcium, which is essential for bone development in both you and your baby. Vitamin D also plays a role in the immune system, muscle function, and cell growth. During pregnancy, it is recommended that women take 600-800 international units (IU) of vitamin D daily.

Food sources of vitamin D include fatty fish such as salmon, tuna, and mackerel, as well as fortified dairy products like milk and yogurt. However, it can be challenging to get enough vitamin D from food alone, especially if you live in a region with limited sun exposure. Vitamin D supplements are often recommended to ensure that you are getting enough of this essential vitamin.

3. Iron

Iron is an essential mineral that is required for the formation of red blood cells, which carry oxygen to your baby. During pregnancy, the body's requirements for iron increase significantly to support the growth and development of the baby. Pregnant women need 27 milligrams (mg) of iron daily, which is almost double the amount needed by non-pregnant women.

Iron deficiency during pregnancy can lead to anemia, a condition in which the body does not have enough red blood cells to carry oxygen to the tissues. Anemia can cause fatigue, weakness, and other health problems for both you and your baby. Therefore, it is essential to ensure that you are getting enough iron in your diet or through supplements.

Food sources of iron include red meat, poultry, fish, beans, and fortified cereals. Iron from animal sources is better absorbed by the body than iron from plant sources. Therefore, if you are a vegetarian or vegan, it is essential to ensure that you are getting enough iron from plant sources or supplements.

4. Vitamin C

Vitamin C is a water-soluble vitamin that plays a role in the immune system and the formation of collagen, a protein that is essential for the development of bones, cartilage, and other connective tissues. Vitamin C also helps the body absorb iron from plant sources. During pregnancy, women need 85 mg of vitamin C daily.

Food sources of vitamin C include citrus fruits, berries, kiwi, melons, tomatoes, peppers, and leafy greens. It is important to note that cooking can destroy some of the vitamin C content in foods, so it is best to eat these foods raw or lightly cooked.

5. Vitamin A

Vitamin A is a fat-soluble vitamin that is essential for vision, immune function, and the development of the heart, lungs, kidneys, and other organs in the baby. However, too much vitamin A can be harmful to the developing fetus, so it is essential to avoid excessive amounts of vitamin A during pregnancy.

Pregnant women should consume no more than 770 micrograms of vitamin A daily. It is important to note that some supplements, especially those derived from fish liver, can contain high levels of vitamin A. Therefore, it is essential to choose a prenatal supplement specifically designed for pregnancy and to consult with your healthcare provider before starting any new supplement regimen.

Food sources of vitamin A include sweet potatoes, carrots, spinach, kale, apricots, and cantaloupe. These foods contain beta-carotene, which is converted to vitamin A in the body and is safe to consume in reasonable amounts during pregnancy.

In addition to these essential vitamins, other vitamins such as vitamin E, vitamin K, and vitamin B12 are also important during pregnancy. It is essential to consume a well-balanced diet that includes a variety of nutrient-rich foods to ensure that you are getting all the necessary vitamins and minerals to support a healthy pregnancy. If you are concerned about your nutrient intake or have a specific dietary restriction, it is always a good idea to consult with your healthcare provider or a registered dietitian.

The Role of Prenatal Supplements

While a healthy diet is the best way to get the necessary vitamins and minerals during pregnancy, prenatal supplements can also play an important role in ensuring that both the mother and the baby are getting all the essential nutrients they need.

Prenatal supplements are specially formulated multivitamins designed for pregnant women, and they typically contain higher levels of key nutrients such as folic acid, iron, and calcium than regular multivitamins. These supplements can help to bridge any gaps in nutrient intake from diet and can provide extra support for the developing fetus.

1. Folic Acid

One of the most critical nutrients found in prenatal supplements is folic acid, which is essential for the proper development of the neural tube in the fetus. Neural tube defects, such as spina bifida, can occur if there is insufficient folic acid intake during pregnancy, which is why it is recommended that all women of childbearing age take a supplement containing at least 400 micrograms of folic acid daily.

2. Iron

Iron is another critical nutrient that is especially important during pregnancy because the mother's blood volume expands significantly to support the growing fetus. Iron is required to produce hemoglobin, a protein found in red blood cells that carries oxygen to the body's tissues. Insufficient iron intake can lead to iron-deficiency anemia, a condition characterized by fatigue, weakness, and shortness of breath.

Pregnant women need 27 milligrams of iron daily, which is almost double the amount needed by non-pregnant women. Prenatal supplements can provide the extra iron needed to meet this requirement, but it is important to note that excessive iron intake can be harmful, so it is essential to follow your healthcare provider's recommended dosage.

3. Calcium

Calcium is necessary for the development of strong bones and teeth in the fetus, and it is also important for the mother's own bone health. Pregnant women need 1,000 milligrams of calcium daily, which can be challenging to achieve through diet alone.

Prenatal supplements can help to ensure that the mother and the baby are getting adequate amounts of calcium, but it is important to note that excessive calcium intake can also be harmful. Taking too much calcium can lead to constipation, kidney stones, and other health problems, so it is essential to follow the recommended dosage and to consult with your healthcare provider before starting any new supplement.

4. Omega-3 Fatty Acids

Omega-3 fatty acids are important for the development of the baby's brain and eyes, and they may also help to prevent preterm labor and postpartum depression. While omega-3 fatty acids can be obtained through diet, many pregnant women do not consume enough of these healthy fats.

Prenatal supplements that contain omega-3 fatty acids can help to ensure that the mother and the baby are getting enough of these essential nutrients. It is important to choose a supplement that is high in the omega-3 fatty acid DHA, which is especially important for fetal brain development.

In addition, while a healthy diet is the best way to get the essential vitamins and minerals during pregnancy, prenatal supplements can help to ensure that both the mother and the baby are getting all the necessary nutrients they need. It is essential to choose a supplement specifically designed for pregnancy, to follow the recommended dosage, and to consult with your healthcare provider before starting any new supplement regimen.

Conclusion:

In conclusion, ensuring that you are getting all the essential vitamins and minerals for a healthy pregnancy is crucial for both you and your baby's health. By eating a well-balanced diet with a variety of nutrient-rich foods and taking a prenatal supplement as recommended by your healthcare provider, you can help to ensure that your body is getting all the necessary nutrients to support a healthy pregnancy.

Remember, every woman and every pregnancy is unique, and your specific nutritional needs may differ from someone else's. Therefore, it is always a good idea to consult with your healthcare provider before making any significant changes to your diet or starting any new supplement regimen.

By taking care of your nutritional needs during pregnancy, you can help to ensure a healthy pregnancy, a healthy baby, and a smooth transition into motherhood.

CHAPTER 5

Managing Pregnancy-Related Symptoms with Nutrition

Pregnancy can be a wonderful and exciting time for women, but it can also be accompanied by a range of uncomfortable symptoms. Nausea, heartburn, constipation, and fatigue are just a few examples of pregnancy-related symptoms that many women experience. While these symptoms can make it challenging to maintain a healthy diet, there are several dietary strategies that can help manage these symptoms and promote good nutrition throughout pregnancy.

1. Nausea

Nausea is a common symptom of early pregnancy, affecting up to 80% of women. This symptom can be particularly challenging as it can make it difficult to consume a healthy, balanced diet. Nausea during pregnancy is thought to be caused by a combination of factors, including hormonal changes, low blood sugar levels, and an increased sense of smell. To manage nausea during pregnancy, try the following dietary strategies:

- Eat small, frequent meals: Eating small, frequent meals throughout the day can help to keep blood sugar levels stable and prevent nausea.

- Avoid triggers: Certain foods or smells can trigger nausea, so it's important to avoid these triggers as much as possible. Common triggers include spicy or greasy foods, strong smells, and foods with strong flavors.
- Eat protein-rich foods: Eating protein-rich foods such as nuts, cheese, or lean meats can help to stabilize blood sugar levels and prevent nausea.
- Stay hydrated: Drinking plenty of water throughout the day can help to prevent dehydration, which can worsen nausea.

2. Heartburn

Heartburn is a common symptom during pregnancy, affecting up to 50% of women. This symptom is caused by the hormonal changes that occur during pregnancy, which can cause the valve between the stomach and esophagus to relax. To manage heartburn during pregnancy, try the following dietary strategies:

- Eat smaller, more frequent meals: Eating smaller, more frequent meals throughout the day can help to prevent the stomach from becoming too full and triggering heartburn.
- Avoid triggers: Certain foods and drinks can trigger heartburn, including spicy or fatty foods, citrus fruits, and carbonated drinks. Avoiding these triggers can help to prevent heartburn.
- Don't lie down after eating: Wait at least two to three hours after eating before lying down. This

can help to prevent stomach acid from flowing back into the esophagus.

3. Constipation

Constipation is a common symptom during pregnancy, affecting up to 40% of women. This symptom is caused by the hormonal changes that occur during pregnancy, which can slow down digestion. To manage constipation during pregnancy, try the following dietary strategies:

- Eat plenty of fiber: Eating foods that are high in fiber can help to promote regular bowel movements. Good sources of fiber include fruits, vegetables, whole grains, and legumes.
- Drink plenty of water: Drinking plenty of water throughout the day can help to soften stool and make it easier to pass.
- Engage in regular physical activity: Regular exercise can help to stimulate the digestive system and promote regular bowel movements.

4. Fatigue

Fatigue is a common symptom during pregnancy, affecting up to 80% of women. This symptom is caused by a combination of factors, including hormonal changes, increased blood volume, and the physical demands of carrying a growing baby. To manage fatigue during pregnancy, try the following dietary strategies:

- Eat a balanced diet: Eating a diet that is rich in whole foods, including fruits, vegetables, lean protein, and healthy fats, can help to maintain steady energy levels throughout the day.

- Avoid processed foods: Processed foods and sugary snacks can cause a rapid spike in blood sugar levels, followed by a crash, which can worsen fatigue.

- Stay hydrated: Dehydration can worsen fatigue, so it is important to drink plenty of water throughout the day. Other hydrating beverages, such as herbal teas or coconut water, can also be helpful.

Food Aversions and Cravings

During pregnancy, many women experience changes in their taste preferences and cravings. While it's important to listen to your body and honor cravings, it's also important to maintain a healthy and balanced diet. Here are some tips for managing food aversions and cravings:

- Experiment with new foods: If you're experiencing food aversions, try experimenting with new foods to find options that are palatable. For example, if you can't tolerate meat, try incorporating plant-based protein sources like lentils or tofu into your diet.

- Choose healthy options: When you experience cravings, try to choose healthier options that still satisfy the craving. For example, if you're craving something sweet, reach for a piece of fruit or a small serving of dark chocolate.

- Keep healthy snacks on hand: To prevent reaching for less healthy options when cravings strike, keep healthy snacks on hand that you enjoy. Some examples include cut-up veggies and hummus, hard-boiled eggs, or trail mix.

In addition to these strategies, it's also important to talk to your healthcare provider about any pregnancy-related symptoms you're experiencing. They can provide guidance on how to manage your symptoms and may recommend additional interventions or treatments if needed.

Overall, managing pregnancy-related symptoms with nutrition can be challenging, but with the right strategies in place, it's possible to maintain a healthy and balanced diet throughout pregnancy. By eating a variety of nutrient-dense foods and listening to your body's needs, you can support your health and the health of your growing baby.

CHAPTER 6

Nutrition for High-Risk Pregnancies

Pregnancy is an exciting and life-changing experience, but it can also be a challenging time for women who have medical conditions or pregnancy complications. Women with high-risk pregnancies require special care and attention to ensure that they and their babies stay healthy throughout the pregnancy.

Nutrition plays a crucial role in managing high-risk pregnancies. A balanced and healthy diet can help to reduce the risk of complications and improve the chances of a successful pregnancy. In this chapter, we will discuss some special considerations for women with medical conditions or pregnancy complications and strategies for managing gestational diabetes, hypertension, and other conditions.

Special Considerations for Women with Medical Conditions or Pregnancy Complications

For women with medical conditions or pregnancy complications, the first step is to work closely with their healthcare provider to develop a plan that ensures their health and the health of their baby. This may involve consulting with specialists, such as an endocrinologist for diabetes or a cardiologist for heart conditions.

In addition to medical management, proper nutrition is essential for women with high-risk pregnancies. Here are some special considerations for women with certain medical conditions:

- Diabetes: Women with diabetes need to carefully manage their blood sugar levels to prevent complications during pregnancy. This may involve frequent blood sugar monitoring and adjusting medication doses as needed. It's also important for women with diabetes to maintain a healthy weight and follow a balanced diet that is low in simple sugars and high in complex carbohydrates, fiber, and protein. Eating small, frequent meals throughout the day can also help stabilize blood sugar levels.

- High blood pressure: Women with high blood pressure may be at risk for developing preeclampsia, a serious condition that can lead to premature delivery and other complications. In addition to medical management, women with high blood pressure should follow a low-sodium diet that is high in potassium, calcium, and magnesium. Regular physical activity, such as walking or swimming, can also help lower blood pressure levels naturally.

- Obesity: Women who are overweight or obese may be at higher risk for complications such as gestational diabetes, hypertension, and preterm delivery. It's important for these women to work with their healthcare provider to develop a plan for healthy weight gain during pregnancy. This may involve following a balanced diet that is high in nutrients but low in calories, as well as engaging in regular physical activity.

Strategies for Managing Gestational Diabetes, Hypertension, and Other Conditions

- Gestational Diabetes: In addition to following a balanced diet, women with gestational diabetes may need to take medication to manage their blood sugar levels. Regular physical activity, such as brisk walking, can also help improve insulin sensitivity and lower blood sugar levels. Women with gestational diabetes may need to monitor their blood sugar levels several times a day and adjust their medication doses as needed.

- Hypertension: Women with hypertension may need to take medication to lower their blood pressure levels. They should also follow a low-sodium diet that is high in potassium, calcium, and magnesium. Regular physical activity can also help lower blood pressure levels naturally. Women with hypertension may need to monitor their blood pressure levels at home and report any changes to their healthcare provider.

- Other Conditions: Women with other medical conditions, such as thyroid disorders or autoimmune disorders, may need to take medication or adjust their medication doses during pregnancy. They should also follow a balanced diet that is high in nutrients and low in processed foods. Regular physical activity can also help improve overall health and reduce the risk of complications.

Conclusion:

Managing a high-risk pregnancy can be challenging, but with proper medical care and nutrition, women can improve their chances of a successful pregnancy outcome. It's important for women with medical conditions or pregnancy complications to work closely with their healthcare provider to develop a plan that meets their unique needs. A balanced diet, regular physical activity, and appropriate medication management can all play a role in ensuring a healthy pregnancy for both the mother and the baby.

CHAPTER 7

Postpartum Nutrition

After giving birth, the focus of new mothers often shifts towards taking care of their baby, and self-care often takes a back seat. However, it is essential to prioritize postpartum nutrition to support the body's recovery and promote healthy breastfeeding. In this chapter, we will discuss the importance of postpartum nutrition and how to maintain a healthy diet and weight post-pregnancy.

Importance of Postpartum Nutrition

Postpartum nutrition is crucial for new mothers because the body goes through significant changes during pregnancy and childbirth. Adequate nutrient intake is necessary for the body's recovery and for supporting breastfeeding. Nutrients such as protein, iron, omega-3 fatty acids, and calcium are essential for postpartum recovery and breastfeeding.

1. Protein

Protein is necessary for tissue repair and muscle growth. During pregnancy, the body produces extra blood, and the uterus and breasts enlarge, which means that protein intake is vital to support these changes. Breastfeeding also requires a significant amount of protein to support milk production. Eating protein-rich foods such as lean meats, fish, poultry, eggs, beans, and legumes is essential for meeting the body's protein needs.

2. Iron

Iron is an essential nutrient that supports the production of hemoglobin, a protein found in red blood cells that carries oxygen to the body's tissues. Women lose a significant amount of blood during childbirth, making it crucial to replenish iron levels. Iron-rich foods such as lean meats, dark leafy greens, nuts, and beans should be consumed regularly. It may also be necessary to take an iron supplement to ensure adequate levels.

3. Omega-3 Fatty Acids

Omega-3 fatty acids are essential for postpartum recovery and breastfeeding as they support brain function and development, reduce inflammation, and may help to prevent postpartum depression. Omega-3 fatty acids are found in fatty fish such as salmon and tuna, as well as chia seeds and flaxseeds. Supplementation may also be necessary to ensure adequate intake.

4. Calcium

Calcium is essential for postpartum recovery as it supports bone health and is necessary for breastfeeding mothers as it supports milk production. Consuming calcium-rich foods such as dairy products, leafy greens, and fortified foods is essential for meeting calcium needs.

Maintaining a Healthy Weight and Balanced Diet Post-Pregnancy

Maintaining a healthy weight and balanced diet post-pregnancy is essential for promoting overall health and wellbeing. Here are some strategies for achieving this:

- Eat a Balanced Diet: A balanced diet consisting of whole grains, lean proteins, healthy fats, and plenty of fruits and vegetables is essential for maintaining a healthy weight post-pregnancy. It is also essential to consume enough calories to support breastfeeding.

- Stay Hydrated: Staying hydrated is essential for postpartum recovery and breastfeeding. Drinking enough water, and other fluids such as milk, herbal tea, and low-sugar beverages can help to prevent dehydration and support milk production.

- Practice Mindful Eating: Practicing mindful eating can help new mothers stay in tune with their body's hunger and fullness cues. Taking time to enjoy meals and snacks, and avoiding distractions while eating can help to prevent overeating.

- Incorporate Physical Activity: Physical activity can help new mothers maintain a healthy weight and promote overall health and wellbeing. Low-impact exercises such as walking, yoga, and swimming can be beneficial for postpartum recovery and can be gradually increased as the body heals.

- Get Enough Sleep: Getting enough sleep is essential for postpartum recovery and for maintaining a healthy weight. New mothers often experience disrupted sleep due to caring for their newborns. Prioritizing sleep when possible can help to reduce stress levels and promote overall health and wellbeing.

In conclusion, postpartum nutrition and maintaining a healthy diet and weight post-pregnancy are essential for promoting overall health and wellbeing. Adequate nutrient intake is necessary for the body's recovery and to support breastfeeding. Eating a balanced diet consisting of whole grains, lean proteins, healthy fats, and plenty of fruits and vegetables is essential for maintaining a healthy weight post-pregnancy. It is also important to stay hydrated, practice mindful eating, incorporate physical activity, and get enough sleep to support postpartum recovery and overall health.

Breastfeeding Nutrition

Breastfeeding is an essential part of postpartum nutrition, and it is essential to prioritize nutrient-dense foods to support milk production. The following are essential nutrients that breastfeeding mothers should consider when planning their meals:

- Water: Drinking enough water is essential for breastfeeding mothers as dehydration can decrease milk supply. Drinking water regularly throughout the day is recommended, and it is essential to listen to the body's thirst cues.

- Protein: Breast milk contains protein, and it is necessary to consume enough protein to support milk production. Eating protein-rich foods such as lean meats, fish, poultry, eggs, beans, and legumes can help meet the body's protein needs.

- Omega-3 Fatty Acids: Omega-3 fatty acids are essential for breastfeeding mothers as they support brain function and development, reduce inflammation, and may help to prevent postpartum depression. Consuming foods rich in omega-3 fatty acids such as fatty fish like salmon and tuna, as well as chia seeds and flaxseeds, can help meet the body's omega-3 fatty acid needs.

- Calcium: Breastfeeding mothers require a significant amount of calcium to support milk production and bone health. Consuming calcium-rich foods such as dairy products, leafy greens, and fortified foods is essential for meeting calcium needs.

- Iron: Iron is essential for breastfeeding mothers as it supports the production of hemoglobin, which carries oxygen to the body's tissues. Breastfeeding mothers may require additional iron as they lose iron through breast milk. Consuming iron-rich foods such as lean meats, dark leafy greens, nuts, and beans can help meet the body's iron needs.

- Vitamins and Minerals: Breastfeeding mothers require a variety of vitamins and minerals to support overall health and wellbeing. Consuming a balanced diet consisting of a variety of fruits, vegetables, whole grains, lean proteins, and healthy fats can help meet the body's vitamin and mineral needs.

In conclusion, postpartum nutrition and maintaining a healthy diet and weight post-pregnancy are essential for promoting overall health and wellbeing. Breastfeeding mothers require additional nutrients to support milk production and should prioritize nutrient-dense foods. It is essential to consume a balanced diet, stay hydrated, practice mindful eating, incorporate physical activity, and get enough sleep to support postpartum recovery and overall health.

Conclusion

Congratulations, you've reached the end of "Optimizing Nutrition During Pregnancy for a Healthy Baby"! We hope that this book has provided you with the knowledge and tools you need to optimize your nutrition during pregnancy and support a healthy pregnancy and baby. As a quick recap, here are some of the key takeaways from the book:

•Proper nutrition during pregnancy is essential for supporting fetal growth and development, reducing the risk of pregnancy complications, and ensuring the mother's health and well-being.

•The key nutrients needed for a healthy pregnancy include protein, iron, folate, calcium, and omega-3 fatty acids, among others.

•Eating a variety of whole foods and avoiding processed foods and excess sugar is important for maintaining optimal nutrition during pregnancy.

•It's also important to pay attention to portion sizes, listen to your body's hunger and fullness cues, and stay hydrated.

•Special considerations may be necessary for women with high-risk pregnancies, such as gestational diabetes and hypertension.

•Postpartum nutrition is also important for a healthy recovery and successful breastfeeding.

As you move forward in your pregnancy journey, we encourage you to continue prioritizing your nutrition and health. Remember, small changes can add up to big benefits for you and your growing baby.

Thank you for reading "Optimizing Nutrition During Pregnancy for a Healthy Baby." We wish you a happy and healthy pregnancy and beyond!